SUGAR DETOX
Defeat Cravings *and* Restore Your Health

Ann Eugene

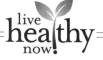

HEALTHY LIVING PUBLICATIONS
Summertown, Tennessee

© 2016 Ann Eugene

All rights reserved. No portion of this book may be reproduced by any means whatsoever, except for brief quotations in reviews, without written permission from the publisher.

Cover and interior design: Scattaregia Design

Healthy Living Publications,
a division of Book Publishing Company
PO Box 99
Summertown, TN 38483
888-260-8458
bookpubco.com

ISBN: 978-1-57067-343-6

> **Disclaimer**
> The information in this book is presented for educational purposes only. It isn't intended to be a substitute for the medical advice of a physician, dietitian, or other health care professional.

Printed in the United States of America

20 19 18 17 16   1 2 3 4 5 6 7 8 9

Library of Congress Cataloging-in-Publication Data

Names: Eugene, Ann, author.
Title: Sugar detox : defeat cravings and restore your health / Ann Eugene.
Description: Summertown, Tennessee : Healthy Living Publications, [2016] | Includes bibliographical references and index.
Identifiers: LCCN 2016013118 (print) | LCCN 2016014579 (ebook) | ISBN 9781570673436 (pbk.) | ISBN 9781570678585 (E-book)
Subjects: LCSH: Sugar-free diet. | Sugar--Health aspects. | Detoxification (Health)
Classification: LCC RM237.85 .E94 2016 (print) | LCC RM237.85 (ebook) | DDC 613.2/8332--dc23
LC record available at http://lccn.loc.gov/2016013118

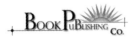

We chose to print this title on responsibly harvested paper stock certified by The Forest Stewardship Council, an independent auditor of responsible forestry practices. For more information, visit https://us.fsc.org.

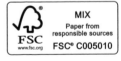

CONTENTS

- **4** Introduction
- **7** Sugar and Its Many Disguises
- **9** Understanding Artificial Sweeteners
- **11** Naturally Occurring Sugars
- **13** A Calorie Isn't Just a Calorie
- **14** Sugar Spikes and the Glycemic Index
- **16** Sugar's Effects on Mental and Physical Health
  - **17** Anxiety
  - **17** Candidiasis
  - **18** Chronic Fatigue Syndrome
  - **19** Depression
  - **19** Fatty Liver Disease
  - **20** Heart Disease
  - **21** Hypothyroidism
  - **22** Irritable Bowel Syndrome
  - **22** Migraine Headaches
  - **23** Obesity
  - **24** Sinusitis
  - **24** Type 2 Diabetes
- **25** An Overview of the Sugar-Detox Plan
- **28** Phase One
- **32** Phase Two
- **36** Phase Three
- **42** Recipes
- **46** Resources
- **46** References
- **47** About the Author

Introduction

- Do you eat even when you're not hungry?
- Are you always thinking about your next meal or snack?
- Do you crave sugary foods and sweets?
- Do you have a family history of diabetes, heart disease, or obesity?
- Does eating cause you distress?
- Do you use food to comfort to you in difficult times?
- Do you use food as a reward?
- Are you currently overweight?
- Do you have excess belly fat?
- Do you eat a healthy diet and exercise regularly but still can't lose weight?
- Do you have heart disease or high blood pressure?
- Are you frequently tired or sluggish?

If you answered yes to even one of the above questions, you've picked up the right guidebook. Chronic maladies such as liver disease, high cholesterol, hypothyroidism, metabolic syndrome, obesity, and type 2 diabetes have become commonplace in our modern culture, plaguing both our personal and public health. Even worse, more and more people are facing these ailments each year. In addition, other prevalent health problems, including anxiety, depression, fatigue, irritable bowel syndrome, migraine headaches, and weight gain, have also become increasingly pervasive.

However, many health experts concur that these conditions as well as numerous others not only can be easily controlled but also prevented. That's because they believe their root cause is a singular enemy: sugar. According to data compiled in 2014 by the market research firm Euromonitor International, the average person in the United States consumes over 126 grams of sugar per day (almost 26 teaspoons). To put this into perspective, that's just about three cans of sugar-sweetened soda. That's also more than double the average sugar intake of all fifty-four countries that were observed by Euromonitor. In addition, it's more than four times what the World Health Organization (WHO) recommends as the daily intake limit: roughly 25 grams of sugar (6 teaspoons) per day for someone of normal weight. The American Heart Association suggests a limit of 6 teaspoons of sugar per day for women, and no more than 9 teaspoons per day for men.

Germany comes in second to the United States, with 103 grams of sugar consumed on average per day. In the Netherlands, about 102.5 grams of sugar is eaten per day; in Ireland, about 97 grams; in Australia, about 95.6 grams; and in Canada, about 89.1 grams. So it shouldn't come as any surprise that all this excess sugar is having a major impact on our health.

But how is this massive quantity of sugar working its way into our diets in the first place? Most of us are aware of the conspicuous high-sugar foods and beverages we consume. But even if you've been trying to limit or omit obvious sources of sugar in your diet, you may not realize that there still is plenty of it lurking in unexpected places. For instance, an average adult's typical daily menu might include a glass of orange juice with breakfast (7½ teaspoons of sugar), store-bought granola sprinkled on yogurt (6 teaspoons of sugar), flavored large latte (12 teaspoons of sugar), and a bowl of pasta with jarred sauce (8 teaspoons of sugar). That equals over 33 teaspoons, and this amount doesn't even take into account all the additional "invisible" sugar that is generally consumed throughout the day from seemingly innocuous sources such as condiments, salad dressings, and even crackers.

According to a report released in 2016 by the British organization Action on Sugar (actiononsugar.org), flavored drinks served by coffee chains such as Starbucks can contain up to 25 teaspoons of sugar per serving. That's almost three times the amount of sugar in one can of cola and about four times the maximum adult daily intake recommended by WHO and the American Heart Association. The research also revealed that a medium Dunkin' Donuts vanilla chai has over 11 teaspoons of sugar, and their hot macchiato contains 7 teaspoons. KFC's mocha contains 15 teaspoons of sugar, while a large mocha at McDonald's has 11 teaspoons.

Why is there so much sugar added to processed foods in the first place? The answer is complicated because manufacturers have found a number of reasons to defend its inclusion. Sugar doesn't only provide sweetness; it also acts as a natural preservative, increases the shelf life and improves the texture of food, enhances the browning of baked goods, boosts the rise of yeasted breads, and balances strong flavors.

As consumers, we generally don't expect to find sugar in foods where it doesn't seem to belong. We all expect, of course, that highly processed sweet items, such as soda, candy, and baked goods, will contain large amounts of sugar. But what about savory crackers, canned peas, seasoned rices, breads, and veggie burgers? Yep, they're all guilty too. The increase of sugar in surprising places has risen rapidly since the 1980s, due in part to the growing supply of low-fat and fat-free processed foods. That's because when fat is removed from a product's formulation, manufacturers often compensate by adding sugar to improve the product's texture and taste.

So what can we do to get off the sugar merry-go-round, reclaim our health, and escape the clutches of the sugar industry and the manufactured products held hostage by it? There are two basic steps to recover health that's been damaged by an overdose of sugar and bounce back from a sugar addiction. The first is the most overt: cut back on sugar as well as processed foods to help thwart further damage. The second step is to replace those nutrient-depleted foods with wholesome, nourishing, healing alternatives. The combination of these tactics is what's known as a sugar detox, a process designed to provide relief from current health symptoms and restore overall wellness. As with any new diet or health regimen, including a sugar detox, be sure to speak with your doctor or health care professional about your plans in advance, especially if you have an existing medical condition.

The good news is that with a sugar detox you won't need to completely overhaul your diet or say good-bye to all your favorite foods (yes, you can even have moderate portions of cake on special occasions). And you won't need to detoxify for longer than ten days. Be aware that as your symptoms diminish, so will your cravings for sugary foods and sweets. By centering your diet on nourishing plant-based proteins, wholesome carbohydrates (even grains!), and beneficial sources of fat, you'll be taking control of your eating habits, building a positive relationship with food, and augmenting your health all at the same time.

A plant-based diet has a long history of helping people restore or maintain good health, stabilize weight, and prevent disease. Although grains and certain sources of concentrated plant-based proteins (such as beans and lentils) are high in carbohydrates, when they're minimally processed, they won't cause spikes in blood sugar the way that refined carbohydrates will. The approach outlined in this guidebook will help ensure that your diet is chock-full of the right combinations and amounts of vegetables, plant-based proteins, whole grains, and other food components to create a healthy, satisfying plan that will work for you.

In the following pages, you'll find all the essential tools to transform your relationship with sugar. You'll learn how to decipher product labels, how to jump-start your diet to eliminate sugar cravings, and how to easily maintain your new style of eating. With this guidebook in hand, you'll be able to restore your health and nix your reliance on that insidious sweet stuff once and for all.

Sugar and Its Many Disguises

One of the reasons sugar frequently slips into our diets unnoticed is because it assumes a variety of identities, some that you're no doubt familiar with: corn syrup, honey, fructose, and molasses, just to name a few. But did you know there are over fifty terms for sugar and that they frequently make an appearance in all kinds of packaged food products and beverages, or that there are more than 250 additional terms that we don't see quite as regularly?

Learning some of the monikers that sugar commonly goes by will give you head start in understanding how to interpret product labels and knowing which products to buy and which ones to avoid.

Agave nectar	Demerara sugar	Malt syrup
Barley malt	Dextran	Malted barley
Beet sugar	Dextrose	extract
Blackstrap molasses	Diatase	Maltodextrin
Brown rice syrup	Ethyl maltol	Maltose
Brown sugar	Evaporated cane juice	Maple sugar
Cane juice	Fructose	Maple syrup
Cane juice crystals	Fruit juice	Molasses
Cane sugar	Fruit juice concentrate	Muscovado
Cane syrup	Galactose	sugar
Caramel	Glucose	Raw sugar
Carob syrup	Glucose-fructose	Refiner's syrup
Castor sugar	Glucose solids	Rice syrup
Coconut sugar	Glucose syrup	Sorbitol
Coconut syrup	Golden syrup	Sorghum syrup
Confectioners' sugar	High-fructose corn	Sucrose
Corn syrup	syrup	Sugar
Corn syrup solids	Honey	Treacle
Crystalline fructose	Icing sugar	Trehalose
Date sugar	Invert sugar	Turbinado sugar
Date syrup	Lactose	Unrefined sugar
	Malt sugar	Yellow sugar

While it's fairly easy to locate the word "sugar" or a basic variation of it on a product label, many packaged foods contain multiple forms of sugar. So even if you find the word "sugar," don't stop there; continue to search for other names that sugar goes by. For example, a popular bottled barbecue sauce contains easy-to-spot "sugar" in its ingredient list, but further reading shows three more types of sugar: blackstrap molasses, glucose-fructose, and honey. A savory plant-based chicken alternative clearly shows organic cane sugar in the label's ingredient list, but then sugar is listed a second time, along with molasses and malted barley extract. A fat-free French dressing contains three entries for sugar: corn syrup and sugar (twice). Not only are these products loaded with sugar, but the latter two hoodwink consumers into thinking they're choosing a healthier option because the product label touts that it's "organic" or "fat-free."

Decoding these ingredient lists might seem overwhelming, but let me assure you that avoiding excess sugar really isn't all that difficult. By simply swapping packaged goods for fresh, plant-based whole foods, you'll discover that you won't really have to do much label reading at all.

Understanding Artificial Sweeteners

Detoxing from sugar doesn't mean a free pass to consume faux sweeteners. Artificial sweeteners, also known as sugar substitutes, nonnutritive sweeteners, and noncaloric sweeteners, are unnatural, manufactured substances that are used as replacements for sugar (sucrose) by consumers and in food manufacturing. There are currently six artificial sweeteners that have been approved by the United States Food and Drug Administration (FDA): acesulfame potassium (also known as acesulfame K and Ace-K), advantame, aspartame, neotame, saccharin, and sucralose. The FDA refers to these as "high-intensity sweeteners" because they are many times sweeter than table sugar.

Although they have been deemed safe for human consumption by the FDA, artificial sweeteners aren't directly sold to consumers in their pure form. The contents of the artificial-sweetener packets at your local coffee shop are mixed with dextrose or maltodextrin to dilute their sweetness so they'll have a taste that's similar to sugar's. Sweet 'N Low (saccharin) and NutraSweet (aspartame) are just two examples of this. But here's something that you won't find on the label: You know that zero calorie count? It's actually not true. Dextrose and maltodextrin both contain calories, but the FDA only requires food manufacturers to list the calories for products if the number is greater than five. If a packet of sweetener contains four calories, those three extra-large "sugar-free" coffees with triple faux sweetener that you sip throughout the day will add up, especially if you're also drinking multiple diet colas and chewing sugarless gum.

It's not just the hidden calories from artificial sweeteners that are problematic, however; research shows that they might contribute to additional health problems. For example, both sugar-sweetened beverages and artificially sweetened beverages have been linked to an increased risk of developing type 2 diabetes and a higher body mass index (BMI). Researchers theorize that artificial sweeteners increase hunger and trigger the body to crave sugar, ultimately resulting in greater caloric intake. These manufactured substances also may suppress the ability to discern the sweetness levels in foods, resulting in the consumption of more sugar to satisfy cravings and inducing a sugar dependency.

Relying on artificial sweeteners to assuage sugar yearnings simply won't do the job. Managing sugar intake and reducing overall consumption will give the body the proper detox it needs—without masking the flavors of real foods. Although right now you might be thinking that a handful of candy could help cut your sugar cravings, just wait—soon, a bowl of ripe berries will be calling your name instead.

Sugar Alcohols

Sugar alcohols (such as D-tagatose, erythritol, glycerol, isomalt, maltitol, mannitol, polydextrose, sorbitol, and xylitol) are additional types of artificial sweeteners. Derived from plant carbohydrates that are chemically altered, sugar alcohols have a lower calorie content than table sugar. However, the chemical-alteration process also results in a substance that cannot be absorbed by the body and that causes a laxative effect upon consumption. When a label states that an item is sugar-free, typically the product contains sugar alcohols.

Stevia and Monk Fruit Extract

Both stevia and monk fruit extract are increasingly being used in food manufacturing to sweeten packaged products. Stevia, *Stevia rebaudiana*, also known as stevioside and sugarleaf, is a tender perennial related to the sunflower plant. Native to parts of South America, stevia has been used for hundreds of years, principally as a sweetener and flavoring agent. It's been estimated that stevia is thirty to three hundred times as sweet as standard table sugar.

Monk fruit, also known as *lo han guo*, is a small round fruit grown in Southeast Asia. The fruit was used for centuries in traditional Eastern medicine as a remedy for colds and digestive disorders. Monk fruit extract, derived from the juice of the crushed fruit, is the latest "sugar-free" addition to the marketplace and is being is used in manufacturing to sweeten a wide range of popular foods and beverages, from protein powders to dairy alternatives. As with similar sugar substitutes, monk fruit is touted as being calorie-free and safe for diabetics, since it won't raise blood sugar levels. Because monk fruit extract can be up to two hundred times as sweet as table sugar, a small amount will pack a powerful punch of sweetness.

Both stevia and monk fruit extract have an aftertaste, which some consumers find off-putting. Additionally, neither product has been approved by the FDA as a regulated sweetener; they have only been given GRAS ("generally recognized as safe") status. A number of research studies are currently underway to explore the effects of stevia and monk fruit extract, but there is much debate on their safety as well as their effectiveness in helping with weight loss or weight management.

Although stevia and monk fruit are derived from plants, they are nevertheless highly processed extractions, not whole foods. Furthermore, because they are incredibly concentrated, they will promote rather than curtail a reliance on sugar and added sweeteners.

Naturally Occurring Sugars

If you've read other books about detoxing from sugar or have family or friends who have done their own detoxifications, you might have heard that fruit is generally forbidden on a sugar detox. All fruits (and even vegetables) contain sugar naturally, although some will have more than others. There are varying approaches to sugar detoxes ranging from including naturally occurring sugars in any amount desired to eliminating them completely.

Many protocols include a strict guideline of consuming no fruit, grains, legumes, and certain vegetables, particularly at the beginning of the detox diet to jump-start the process. In this guidebook, the approach outlined in phase two (see page 32) falls into that category. However, unlike other methods, the consumption of some nutrient-dense foods, such as legumes and larger portions of vegetables, is encouraged in order to meet nutritional needs. A sugar detox doesn't need to be overly restrictive and shouldn't cause frustration. Instead, the goal is to reduce reliance on sugar and resolve its resultant effects on health.

Some sugar-detox plans are aligned with low-carb diets, but the plant-based protocol outlined in this guidebook doesn't fall into that category. Don't confuse a sugar detox with a low-carb diet, which restricts carbohydrate consumption and encourages replacing high-carb foods with greater amounts of fat and protein.

The word "carbohydrate" is often misunderstood and lobbed about rather loosely among dieters and health proponents. It's frequently used as an umbrella term to encompass grains, legumes, and white potatoes. In actuality there are three main groups of carbohydrates: starches (complex carbohydrates), fiber, and sugar.

Foods that are naturally high in starch include legumes (fresh and dried peas, beans, and lentils), grains (such as barley, oats, rice, and wheat), and foods made with grains (such as bread, crackers, and pasta).

Fiber is only available in plant foods, such as vegetables, fruits, nuts, whole grains, and legumes. Most of this dietary fiber passes through the intestines undigested. Fiber is beneficial to health because it helps improve regularity and curb constipation and contributes to a sense of fullness and satiety after eating. Fiber is also credited with helping to reduce cholesterol levels.

A sugar detox based on whole foods, as outlined in this guidebook, is designed to help you reduce or eliminate added dietary sugar while providing guidance and support in selecting wholesome, minimally processed foods that are naturally low in sugar but rich in vital nutrition and healthy starches and fiber. The right foods are what make this sugar detox effective, and knowing which ones to select will make this protocol work for you.

A Calorie Isn't Just a Calorie

You might be familiar with the old adage "a calorie is a calorie." Despite the prevalence of this saying, it isn't really true. To demonstrate the differences, table 1 provides a breakdown of three different food examples, each containing approximately 140 calories:

Table 1. Nutrient comparison of foods with comparable calories

Food	Sugar (added or naturally occurring), in grams	Fiber, in grams	Fat, in grams	Protein, in grams
¼ cup jelly beans	27	0	0	2
½ large apple, plus 1 tablespoon almond butter	12	3	8	5
23 stalks celery	15	14	1	7

If it were true that a calorie is a calorie, then any of the three entries in table 1 would be an equally smart snack choice, but that simply isn't the case. Although the apple and celery are clearly healthier options than the jelly beans, it's actually the apple that comes out on top. The apple, combined with the almond butter, provides a better balance of nutrients, and the unsaturated fat in the almond butter will help stave off hunger longer.

With all of their added sugar and lack of fat, fiber, and protein, those jelly beans just aren't going to satisfy. In fact, they are going to spike your blood sugar, and ultimately make you hungrier—especially for something sweet. Conversely, the fat, fiber, and protein in the apple and almond butter will prevent a sugar spike that would inevitably drive that hunger into overdrive a short time later.

Sugar Spikes and the Glycemic Index

You've probably heard the terms "sugar spike" and "sugar crash," but you might not know exactly what they mean. These terms often coincide with talk about the glycemic index, which is the underpinning of popular diets of yesteryear, such as the Atkins diet and the South Beach Diet. The glycemic index (GI) is a measure of how quickly carbohydrates (such as sugar) raise blood sugar levels. The GI is measured on a scale of up to 100, with glucose (a simple sugar) having a value of 100. Foods that are high on the glycemic index cause a sharper rise in blood sugar. It is important to note that what makes them high on the scale is not always the type of food that's consumed: the method of cooking, length of cooking time, and level of freshness or ripeness all can influence glycemic-index outcomes.

Most GI tables include an extra breakdown for the glycemic load. The glycemic load connects how much sugar a food contains to the rate of the body's absorption of that sugar. This helps do away with the controversy that all "high-sugar" (but nevertheless nutritious) foods should be avoided. Carrots, for example, fall into this often misunderstood category, and people who consume a typical low-carbohydrate diet frequently avoid carrots because they are high on the glycemic index. However, the overall amount of sugar consumed in a serving of carrots is in reality quite small, resulting in a low glycemic load. Consequently, carrots can and should be eaten freely, even on a low-carb diet.

It isn't necessary to memorize the entire glycemic index and load value of foods to successfully follow a sugar detox, but it is important to be aware of specific foods that don't fall where you might have anticipated them to. Most sources use three ratings for the glycemic index: Low (0 to 55), Medium (56 to 69), and High (70 and above). The World's Healthiest Foods website (whfoods.com) includes a fourth group, Very Low, for foods that have a GI rating of 20 or below. The recommended diet that's outlined in this guidebook uses these groups as a starting point. For searchable databases of the GI measurement for numerous foods, see Resources, page 46. Table 2, below, provides a general overview of common food items and their glycemic index and glycemic load values per serving.

Table 2. GI values and glycemic load per serving of common foods

Food	Glycemic index rating	Glycemic load (per serving)
Russet potato, baked (150 g)	111	33
Corn flakes (30 g)	93	23
White rice (150 g)	89	43
Oatmeal, instant (250 g)	83	30
Rice cakes (25 g)	82	17
Potato, white, boiled (150 g)	82	21
Watermelon (120 g)	72	4
Whole wheat bread (30 g)	71	9
Sweet potato (150 g)	70	22
Cola (250 mL)	63	16
Banana, ripe (120 g)	62	16
Spaghetti, soft (180 g)	58	26
Oatmeal, old-fashioned rolled oats (250 g)	55	13
Quinoa (150 g)	53	13
Orange juice, pure (250 mL)	50	12
Brown rice (150 g)	50	16
Spaghetti, al dente (180 g)	46	22
Dates, dried (60 g)	42	18
Apple (120 g)	39	6
Chickpeas (garbanzo beans) (150 g)	38	9
Tomato juice (250 mL)	38	4
Black beans (150 g)	30	7
Lentils (150 g)	29	5
Cashews (50 g)	27	3
Peanuts (50 g)	7	0

Note the importance of how cooking the same food two different ways can affect the outcome. Overcooking pasta, for example, increases the sugar content, and baking a potato results in a higher GI number than it does for potatoes that are boiled. Similarly, the way a food is processed, as with instant oatmeal versus old-fashioned rolled oats, makes a dramatic difference in the GI level and glycemic load. Of course all of this can be confusing and overwhelming, which is why simply focusing on minimally processed whole foods can help you easily achieve success in your sugar detox without unnecessary frustration.

Eating foods with a lower glycemic index will not only help keep your blood sugar stable but will also assist with reducing "bad" cholesterol, regulating your appetite, and lowering your risk of type 2 diabetes and heart disease. The primary components of a low-sugar diet include nonstarchy vegetables, high-quality plant-based protein, and healthy fats, which are anti-inflammatory and will keep you satiated longer. These are secondarily supplemented with starchy vegetables, whole grains, and fruits. If you're eating the right foods, you won't have to worry about how much of them you eat; quality surpasses quantity in importance.

Sugar's Effects on Mental and Physical Health

Whether you have a clear diagnosis of a health problem related to sugar, have a physical or mental illness that may be exacerbated by excess sugar, want to improve your overall health, or feel that you are "addicted" to sugar, you can find help and support by following the protocols in this guidebook. Although the following descriptions and recommendations are derived from current literature and studies on the effects of sugar on health, always speak with your doctor before making changes to your diet, especially if you have been diagnosed with a medical condition or are taking any medications.

Anxiety

Too much sugar can make us feel tense, jittery, keyed up, and on edge. Have you ever overindulged and ended up with a case of the sugar shakes? Excess sugar taxes the adrenal glands, which secrete adrenaline to help us cope with stressful situations and initiates the "flight or fight" response. Too much sugar at a pop can cause what's commonly called an "adrenaline rush." If you suffer from anxiety or chronic stress, this abundance of adrenaline can push you into panic mode. Further, if you're choosing sugar-laden sweets over healthy whole foods, you might be missing out on essential nutrients, especially those that have a relaxing effect on the body, such as magnesium and B-complex vitamins.

Many foods suggested in phases two (see page 32) and three (see page 36) of the sugar detox, such as almonds, dark leafy greens, flaxseeds, soy products, and walnuts, are very good sources of B-complex vitamins. The amino acid theanine, which stimulates a state of deep relaxation and mental alertness and assists in releasing the "feel good" chemicals serotonin and dopamine, is found in green tea, which is also recommended in phases two and three. Try to incorporate all of these into your daily diet.

Candidiasis

Candidiasis is a fungal infection caused by an overgrowth of yeasts that belong to the genus *Candida*. Candidiasis that develops in the mouth or throat is called "thrush," or oropharyngeal candidiasis. Candidiasis in the vagina is commonly referred to as a "yeast infection." Invasive candidiasis occurs when *Candida* species enter the bloodstream and spread throughout the body. Although this yeast is normally found in small amounts in the human body, certain medicines (such as antibiotics) and health problems (such as diabetes or digestive disorders) can cause more yeast to grow, particularly in warm, moist areas of the body. Symptoms can range from mild discomfort to serious and painful complications.

Yeast, including *Candida*, feed on sugar, so a sugar-laden diet can also be the cause of candidiasis. Furthermore, a diet heavy in sugar can aggravate the condition and its symptoms by encouraging the yeast to thrive and multiply. If you know or suspect that candidiasis is the cause of your symptoms, you may want to stay on phase two (page 32) until you experience a substantial improvement in your condition. This will decrease the risk of a setback when you begin to reintroduce foods in phase three. Once phase three begins, add new foods gradually to test how your body responds to them.

Chronic Fatigue Syndrome

Chronic fatigue syndrome (CFS) is commonly underdiagnosed as well as misdiagnosed. Described as a persistent fatigue that does not go away, combined with pain and severe brain fog, it is thought to be caused by a malfunction of the hypothalamus, which regulates the body's temperature, hormones, blood flow, blood pressure, and other homeostatic systems. For people with chronic fatigue syndrome, more rest doesn't result in more energy. Instead, people with chronic fatigue syndrome usually experience a downward spiral into feeling increasingly unwell.

When chronic fatigue sets in, sufferers often turn to unhealthy food choices to give them a lift. Whether it's a sugary cola (or two) as a pick-me-up, fast-food dinners loaded with refined carbohydrates when there's no energy left to cook, or a vending-machine snack just to make it through the workday, once the cycle begins, health gets depleted further and faster. These non-nutritive, sugar-laden, refined foods cause internal stress and inflammation, from the bowels to the sinuses, and affect overall health, making CFS sufferers more susceptible to infection and further fueling their illness.

Ensure that during phases two and three of the sugar detox that you're fueling your body with enough calories, fat, and protein from nutrient-dense whole foods so you have the energy you need to recuperate. Make your fatigue your focus, with the goal to feel better overall before you tackle other health issues.

Depression

As with anxiety (see page 17), symptoms of depression may be aggravated by nutritional deficiencies. In addition, other illnesses that may accompany depression, such as chronic fatigue syndrome (see page 18) or obesity (see page 23), often result in lethargy and inactivity. Many studies show that exercise is associated with lower incidences of depression and that physical activity and working out may even help to treat the condition.

Omega-3 fatty acids, found primarily in certain fish and their oils and particular types of nuts and seeds, play a key role in brain function and decreasing symptoms of depression. However, these essential fatty acids are often in short supply for people following plant-based diets. There are three types of omega-3 fatty acids: ALA (alpha-linolenic acid, found in both plant- and animal-based foods), EPA (eicosapentaenoic acid, found mainly in fish), and DHA (docosahexaenoic acid, found mainly in fish and sea vegetables). The body can convert ALA to EPA and DHA, although large amounts of ALA are required for the latter. Many nutrition experts recommended that people on a plant-based diet take a DHA supplement, but because too much omega-3 fatty acids can cause bleeding and bruising, it would be best to speak to your health care professional before starting on this type of supplementation. In the meantime, phases two and three of the sugar detox encourage the consumption of an abundance of omega-3-rich plant foods, such as walnuts and flaxseeds, and discourage the consumption of fats with a high omega-6 content, such as corn oil and soy oil.

Fatty Liver Disease

Non-alcoholic fatty liver disease (NAFLD) is a widespread health problem in the United States, affecting over 25 percent of the population. In addition, it is rapidly becoming the most common liver disease worldwide, with the prevalence of NAFLD in the general population of Western countries ranging from 20 to 30 percent. The prevalence of NAFLD is 80 to 90 percent in obese adults and 30 to 50 percent in patients with diabetes. The prevalence of NAFLD among children is 3 to 10 percent, but it rises to 40 to 70 percent among obese children. Moreover, pediatric NAFLD increased from about 3 percent a decade ago to 5 percent today.

NAFLD is the buildup of extra fat in liver cells that is not caused by alcohol. It's normal for the liver to contain some fat. However, if fat comprises more than 5 to 10 percent of the liver's weight, the liver is considered fatty (steatosis). NAFLD tends to develop in people who are overweight or obese or who have diabetes, high cholesterol, or high triglycerides. Lack of exercise and poor eating habits, including the consumption of excess sugar, have been linked to these conditions, as well as to NAFLD.

NAFLD often has no symptoms, but when symptoms do occur, they may include fatigue, weakness, weight loss, loss of appetite, nausea, abdominal pain, yellowing of the skin and eyes (jaundice), itching, fluid buildup, swelling of the legs (edema) and abdomen (ascites), and mental confusion. The more severe form of NAFLD is called non-alcoholic steatohepatitis (NASH), which causes the liver to swell and become damaged. NASH is one of the leading causes of cirrhosis in adults in the United States.

Recommended treatments for NAFLD include losing weight if you are overweight or obese, lowering your cholesterol and triglyceride levels, controlling your diabetes, exercising, and avoiding alchohol. Eating a healthy diet, along with exercising regularly, may help prevent liver damage from starting in the first place or could reverse it in the early stages. If you have NAFLD, be sure to regularly visit a doctor who specializes in the liver and discuss your sugar-detox plans, including how long you should stay on phase two of the detox diet.

Heart Disease

Many diseases and illnesses cause excess strain on the heart. However, heart disease itself can be caused by something as simple as too much added sugar in the diet. According to a 2014 study published in the *Journal of the American Medical Association Internal Medicine*, people who consumed 17 to 21 percent of calories from added sugar had a 38 percent higher risk of dying from heart disease compared to those who consumed only 8 percent. This was the first study that specifically linked heart disease and sugar, irrespective of other health factors, such as high blood pressure, high cholesterol, and obesity.

Heart disease is often quite preventable. While on phases two and three of the sugar detox, you can further reduce your susceptibility to heart disease through additional healthy lifestyle choices, such as not smoking, avoiding alcohol, and being physically active.

Hypothyroidism

Thyroid hormones play an essential role in a variety of metabolic and developmental processes in the human body. Hypothyroidism, also called underactive thyroid, is a condition in which the thyroid gland does not make enough thyroid hormone. The thyroid gland, located at the front of the neck, is an important organ of the endocrine system. The thyroid makes hormones that control the way every cell in the body uses energy.

Thyroid disorders have become increasingly linked with diabetes and obesity. This is because stable blood sugar levels depend on healthy thyroid function, and a healthy thyroid depends on stable blood sugar levels. Excess dietary sugar taxes the pancreas by forcing it to secrete additional insulin to balance blood glucose levels, a process that can eventually cause cells to lose their ability to respond to insulin, known as insulin resistance. It can also damage the adrenal and thyroid glands and cause thyroid hormone production to fail.

If you have hypothyroidism combined with type 2 diabetes, it is doubly important to maintain steady blood sugar. Follow the protocols in phases two and three, and make sure you are prepared with wholesome snacks to consume every few hours. Strive for five or six smaller meals throughout the day if three large meals and small snacks produce undesirable symptoms.

Irritable Bowel Syndrome

Irritable bowel syndrome (IBS) refers to a functional digestive disorder that typically involves a broad range of symptoms, including gas, bloating, diarrhea and/or constipation, and abdominal pain, without evidence of disease or structural damage (as there is with inflammatory bowel diseases, such as Crohn's disease or ulcerative colitis). There is no known cause or cure for IBS. However, many other conditions, such as food sensitivities, candidiasis (see page 17), small intestinal bacterial overgrowth (SIBO), and leaky gut syndrome can exacerbate symptoms of IBS. Not only can excess dietary sugar contribute to the development of these conditions, but it can also worsen IBS by irritating the digestive tract and triggering or worsening symptoms.

It is important to follow the guidelines in the sugar-detox protocols while also selecting foods that don't aggravate your symptoms. Some nutritious foods, such as dark leafy greens, can be enjoyed in abundance on the sugar detox, but people with IBS may find them difficult to digest. Healthful fats, such as olive oil, are generally recommended, but not when you're in the throes of severe diarrhea. You may need to make modifications to the diet that work for your body, especially if you're in the midst of a flare-up, and take note of your symptoms along the way. As mentioned on page 10, it is important to avoid consuming sugar alcohols; this is particularly critical for people with IBS. Sugar alcohols not only have a laxative effect, but they also encourage unfriendly gut bacteria and yeasts to proliferate.

Migraine Headaches

There is no single cause of migraine headaches, and their numerous triggers are still not fully understood. However, there is a known association between migraine headaches and nutrient deficiencies, as well as chronic inflammation. If you believe that one of these is the cause of your migraines, decreasing sugar might be the solution. In addition, being deficient in B-complex vitamins and/or magnesium can play a role in migraines and headaches in general.

If you suffer from migraines, reduce or eliminate your reliance on high-sugar snacks. Also monitor your diet, exercise habits, and stress levels to determine their effects on the incidence and frequency of your migraines.

Obesity

Obesity is one of the most pervasive health consequences of a high-sugar diet. This is significant because obesity is one of leading causes of preventable death. Obesity-related conditions include heart disease, stroke, type 2 diabetes and certain types of cancer. You may be thinking that this isn't a problem for you, and that might be true . . . for now. According to the Centers for Disease Control and Prevention (cdc.gov), about 70 percent of adult Americans in 2014 were overweight, and about 35 percent were classified as obese. These numbers don't account for people who are "apple-shaped" and carry a little extra weight around the middle. Often referred to as belly fat, this additional layer of adipose tissue is exactly what increases the risk of prediabetes and metabolic syndrome, which can snowball into a host of other health problems, including full-blown type 2 diabetes, heart disease, and stroke. The Centers for Disease Control and Prevention (CDC) estimates the annual medical cost of obesity in the United States was $147 billion in 2008; the medical costs for people who are obese were $1,429 higher than those of normal weight.

It's not just adults who are affected by obesity. In 2014 the CDC noted that obesity more than doubled in children and quadrupled in adolescents over the past thirty years. In 2012 it reported that more than one-third of children and adolescents in the United States were obese or overweight.

Don't be tempted to stay in phase two (page 32) of the detox beyond what is necessary, as long as your cravings and symptoms decrease or disappear entirely. If you are currently overweight or obese, you will not lose all your weight in the allotted three to ten days of the detox, and that's okay. What's important is that you are steadily losing weight on phase three (page 36), your cravings are under control, and you have improved other aspects of your lifestyle, such as increasing your physical activity. You will still be successfully detoxing from sugar in a healthy way that will be easy to continue and maintain.

Sinusitis

Sugar-aggravated candidiasis (page 17) and chronic inflammation can contribute to or cause sinusitis. Excessive bacteria worsen inflammation, and both candidiasis and inflammation can increase swelling and block the nasal passages and sinuses, often resulting in infection. Once infection sets in, antibiotics are typically prescribed. However, this sets up the perfect storm for what's known as antibiotic syndrome, a cyclic pattern of infection and antibiotic use. That's because antibiotics destroy not only harmful bacteria but also beneficial bacteria that help ward off infection, inflammation, and bacterial and yeast overgrowth. Regular antibiotic use also creates a host of additional problems by causing bacterial imbalances throughout the body, including in the digestive tract.

The best cure for chronic sinusitis is to avoid getting it in the first place. By decreasing your overall sugar intake, you will impede opportunistic bacteria and yeast from proliferating and lessen their chances of establishing an overgrowth or causing inflammation in your body.

Type 2 Diabetes

Although type 2 diabetes is not specifically caused by eating too much sugar, excessive sugar consumption frequently leads to obesity, and obesity greatly increases the risk of type 2 diabetes. Lifestyle factors and genetic predisposition are also believed to contribute to the risk of type 2 diabetes, but it's equally possible that poor health choices are learned and passed down among families, rather than inherited via genetics. Overconsumption of sugar not only contributes to type 2 diabetes by helping to pack on pounds, but it also increases blood glucose levels and pushes the pancreas into overdrive so it can make extra insulin to regulate the levels.

Designed to decrease or eliminate your risk of type 2 diabetes, phases two and three of the sugar detox will help regulate your blood sugar by incorporating safe, nutritious foods based on the glycemic index and glycemic load. If you have already been diagnosed with type 2 diabetes, you may have to alter the way you currently manage your disease via diet. That's because many diabetic-friendly products, such diet soda and "sugar-free" candies, are not recommended on this detox.

An Overview of the Sugar-Detox Plan

This guidebook outlines a sugar detox that's suitable for people dealing with any of the sugar-related maladies listed on pages 17 through 24, as well as for people who have a clean bill of health but are consuming more sugar per day than is recommended. Even if disease isn't manifesting in your body right now, a reduced-sugar diet will ensure that your good health continues for the rest of your life. The detox will also help you better understand how your body operates in terms of fueling your physical activity or combating cravings.

Physical Activity

The Centers for Disease Control and Prevention recommends that adults ages eighteen to sixty-four participate in muscle-strengthening activities two or more days a week and get at least one of the following:

- 2 hours and 30 minutes of moderate-intensity aerobic activity every week
- 1 hour and 15 minutes of vigorous-intensity aerobic activity every week
- an equivalent mix of moderate and vigorous-intensity aerobic activity every week

While you're on the sugar detox (and even after you've finished it), try to stick close to these guidelines. If you engage in very high-intensity physical activity, you may need to modify the suggested food intake (particularly the carbohydrate intake) outlined in this guidebook to meet your increased needs. This may include consuming simple sugars during marathon training or bumping up the number of servings of legumes to get you through a physically demanding full-time job. If that describes your situation, use phase two as a general guideline to eliminate added sugar in your diet (such as that handful of cookies after a long run) while continuing with your own tried-and-true dietary tactics (such as having sports drinks during lengthy runs in hot weather) to fulfill your nutrient needs. Focus on high-quality foods to meet your individual requirements and rid yourself of sugar cravings.

Coping with Cravings

A craving is defined as a deep yearning or need. A food craving often arises to satisfy an emotional need, commonly stemming from stress or anxiety. These cravings take hold in the areas of the brain responsible for sensing pleasure and establishing memory.

Eating sugar creates a natural high, releasing endorphins that are temporarily calming and relaxing, but these pleasant sensations are fleeting. Sugar in the form of simple carbohydrates is quickly absorbed into the bloodstream, causing blood sugar levels to rise almost immediately. Insulin is then released and sugar enters the cells, leaving the bloodstream and helping the body return to its normal state. Because the enjoyable feelings brought on by the sugar dissipate quickly, we end up wanting more sugar so we can experience them again. This sets up an endless cycle:

cravings→sugar consumption to quell the cravings→sugar high →physical or emotional crash (when the effects of the sugar wear off)→more cravings

The protocols in this guidebook will help you get rid of your cravings and break the cycle once and for all. By following the balanced, pragmatic approach outlined in the next sections, you will still be able to consume added sugars in moderation while tuning in to your body's needs and feeding it the nutrition it requires.

The Diet

Even if you don't think you actually consume that much added sugar, don't underestimate the ways that sugar in all its manifestations worms its way into food. Sure, you might not be noshing on a doughnut and a two-sugar coffee from the drive-thru on the way to work each morning, but sugar is still sugar. That handful of trail mix, cup of yogurt, peanut butter and jelly sandwich, fruit salad, blueberry smoothie—all nutritious options—can still add up to over 30 teaspoons of sugar! That's a far cry from the limit of 6 teaspoons of added sugar recommended by respected health organizations, such as the American Heart Association and World Health Organization.

Getting Started

The solution to reducing sugar intake lies in consuming a whole-foods diet. A diet centered on minimally processed plant foods that are as close as possible to the way nature packaged them provides less opportunity for sugar to sneak in. The sugar detox described in this guidebook is broken down into three phases to make the process as easy as possible.

Phase one helps you take a new approach to your relationship with food. This is the time you'll clean out your refrigerator and pantry, learn how to read labels more carefully, find substitutions for your favorite sugar-laden foods, and adopt the best mindset to proceed to phase two.

Phase two is when the dietary changes begin. During this phase you'll jump into the detoxification process, work on those cravings, and reset your metabolism. This phase is a bit stringent, but it only needs to last three to ten days, depending on what works best for you. Follow phase two for three days if you eat a relatively unprocessed diet or have done a sugar detox in the past, or if your health professional recommends that you stay on the detox just a short time. Follow the detox for four to seven days if you don't see relief from cravings after three days, need a little more time to adjust your mindset, or are still feeling symptomatic. Continue phase two for eight to ten days if this is the first time you've done a sugar detox. If after eight days your cravings and symptoms disappear, move on to phase three; otherwise, continue phase two for a full ten days.

Once you have completed phases one and two, you can transition to phase three. This phase is designed for maintenance. During phase three you will gradually reintroduce foods that weren't permitted in phase two and learn how to balance your diet and lifestyle.

Bear in mind that there are no hard and fast rules. You don't have to start over if you eat something that's "off limits" in one of the phases. The process is designed to work with you at your current level; just be sure not to move on to the next phase until you feel ready to. Let's begin!

Phase One

Success with any sugar detox relies on the power of knowledge. By having a bit of pantry proficiency, knowing how to properly restock your fridge and freezer, understanding the truth about product labels, learning how to cook tasty and nutritious meals, and choosing the best substitutions, you will be able to recover and maintain good health.

Overhauling the Pantry and Fridge

Clearing out the pantry is comparable to detoxifying the body: the end result will make you feel lighter, healthier, and cleaner. If processed foods are a mainstay of your diet, then getting them out of your house is the first place to start. Your kitchen should be a safe zone––a place that's free of temptations that might undermine your detox efforts. Save any special treats for times when it's really worth it, such as having a glass of wine with friends, getting a celebration dessert at your favorite restaurant, or enjoying a large no-butter popcorn at the movie theater on date night. Follow these steps and you'll get your detox off to a great start:

1. Have large box and a trash bag available. There are two places the foods you're clearing out should go: the local food bank or the trash. The box is where to put the items for the food bank. The trash bag is for perishables that are past their prime and for expired items.

2. Read labels. Twice. Retain items that haven't yet expired and only contain whole, natural ingredients. In general, if you don't recognize an ingredient or can't pronounce it, or if an item contains preservatives, food coloring, sugar in any form (see page 7), or artificial sweetener (see page 9), it should be moved to the box or trash bag.

3. Replenish with the right foods. Once you clear out your cupboards, fridge, and freezer, you can start restocking with the right choices. The easiest way to approach a sugar detox as well as a low-sugar diet is to focus on whole foods that contain just one ingredient—the food itself. For packaged products, seek items that are free of any kind of sugar (see page 7) and have very few ingredients.

When purchasing packaged foods, take a look at the serving size listed on the label. Make sure that size seems reasonable to you, because most packaged items have serving sizes that are much smaller than what the average person eats at a sitting. Check the number of calories per serving along with the amount of fat, protein, carbohydrates, and sodium. Look under the "carbohydrate" heading for fiber. Aim for consuming 5 to 10 grams of fiber per meal, and between 25 and 30 grams of total fiber per day. Also under the "carbohydrate" heading will be "sugar." Of course, you'll want to seek out products that contain as little added sugar as possible (preferably no more than 8 grams). If no sugar is listed in the ingredient breakdown, any sugar on the nutrition panel would come from natural sources, such as fruit. And although sodium intake is not directly related to detoxing from sugar, it is related to overall health. Any packaged foods in your pantry should contain less than 400 milligrams of sodium per serving.

> **No Sugar Added versus Sugar-Free**
>
> What's the difference between "no sugar added" and "sugar-free" on a product label? These listings can make choosing the right foods a challenge. According to the US Food and Drug Administration, "no sugar added" can only be used on a product label if no sugar or sugar-containing ingredient is used during processing. However, this doesn't mean a product is sugar-free. Packaged frozen mango slices, for example, may have no sugar added, but the product still contains naturally occurring sugar in the mangoes.
>
> A product that touts "sugar-free" on the label must contain less than 0.5 grams of sugar per serving. This includes both naturally occurring sugar and ingredients that contain sugar.
>
> Because packaged products may contain artificial sweeteners, hidden sugar, and other undesirable ingredients, it is wise to always read labels closely and carefully each time you purchase an item. Formulations and product ingredients often change over time, and most manufacturers don't note that overtly on the package.

Cooking Equals Success

People who cook for themselves have already taken a big leap toward a healthier diet. Cooking doesn't have to be complicated, inconvenient, or expensive. It can actually be enjoyable and rewarding. The benefit of preparing your own food rather than purchasing processed items is that you know exactly what you're eating. Of course, some minimally processed packaged foods with limited ingredients can be good for us: unsweetened, natural peanut butter, dried herbs and spices, flavorful oils, and tangy vinegars, for example, can add zest, richness, and excitement even to very simple meals.

Simple Swaps

Learning some nutritious substitutions for off-limits foods can make a sugar detox relatively painless. Try replacing your midafternoon latte with an invigorating herbal tea, such as soothing peppermint or ginger. Ditch that bag of candy for a cup of unsweetened nondairy yogurt. Or snack on a handful of homemade granola (see page 42) instead of a bowl of cornflakes. Didn't I tell you it could be painless?

Table 3, below, lists some common high-sugar foods and possible alternatives for you try as replacements.

Table 3. Foods high in sugar/high glycemic load and simple substitutions

High-sugar foods	Low-sugar alternatives
Breakfast cereals	Anything Goes Granola (page 42)
Canned tomato soup	Classic Tomato Soup (page 43)
Dry-roasted nuts	Crunchy Chickpeas (page 45); raw or roasted nuts or seeds without additives, except a little sea salt or oil
Jam, jelly, and preserves	Mashed fresh fruit, such as banana or strawberries
Ketchup	Salsa; tomato paste, plain or with a dash of cider vinegar
Mashed potatoes	Mashed cauliflower; mashed root vegetables; whole-grain polenta
Mayonnaise	Mashed avocado
Microwave popcorn	Home-popped popcorn (using a hot-air popper or the stove top) seasoned with extra-virgin olive oil or coconut oil, a spritz of tamari or a light sprinkle of sea salt, and a dusting of nutritional yeast
Pancakes with syrup	Pancakes made with whole-grain flours and topped with fresh fruit or berries
Salad dressing	Extra-virgin olive oil and flavorful vinegars (balsamic, cider, and wine vinegars)
Veggie dogs	Smoked tofu
White rice	Brown rice; quinoa

Phase Two

Phase two will help you work on cravings and reset your metabolism. It is strict, and it might be a little rough going, especially at first, but it only lasts three to ten days (see pages 27–28). Once you feel that you are less symptomatic than before you started the detox, and your cravings for sugar have disappeared, you'll be ready to move to phase three.

How Strict Is Strict?

The word "strict" is used loosely here. In fact, you've chosen an approach that is much more flexible and forgiving than most other sugar detoxes, which often call for nixing sugar in all its forms, including healthy carbohydrates, such as whole grains and legumes, not only during the first phases but for maintenance as well. This protocol includes these foods and has just a short list of foods to avoid.

This might seem complicated but it really isn't. After all, you have the basics outlined right here. First, stock your pantry, refrigerator, and freezer using the foods listed in table 4. Then follow the simple guideline in table 6 for your daily meals and snacks.

Table 4. Foods to enjoy in phase two

Type of Food	Foods Allowed	Notes
Beverages (no sugar added)	Coffee, sparkling water, low-sodium club soda, unsweetened nondairy beverages, unsweetened tea	Any sweetened or artificially sweetened beverages are off limits during this phase. If you regularly indulge in sodas, juices, and other sugary beverages, take ten days to wean yourself off them before starting on phase two of the detox.
Fruits	Avocado, coconut, lemon, lime	Fruits are limited because of their high sugar content.

Grains, whole	Amaranth, long-grain brown rice, Kamut, quinoa, sorghum, spelt, steel-cut oats, old-fashioned rolled oats, teff, wild rice	Have up to 1 cup of cooked whole grains twice a day.
Legumes	All legumes (beans, lentils, and peas)	Have up to ½ cup of cooked legumes per meal.
Nuts and Sugar-Free Nut Butters	Almonds, brazil nuts, cashews, coconut, hazelnuts, peanuts, pecans, pistachios, walnuts	Look for nut butters that only contain nuts and salt. Limit nuts to a 1-ounce serving about three times a day and choose from a wide variety of nuts.
Oils	Avocado oil, coconut oil, extra-virgin olive oil, flaxseed oil, nut oils (almond, macadamia, walnut), pumpkin seed oil, sesame oil	There are no maximums for fats and oils on the detox, but be mindful of how much you are taking in. About one-eighth of your meals and snacks should contain some sort of fat, which includes avocado, coconut, seeds, and nuts.
Seeds and Seed Butters (no sugar added)	Chia, flax, hemp, pumpkin, sesame, sunflower, tahini	Look for seed butters that only include seeds and salt. Limit seeds to a 1-ounce serving about three times a day and choose from a wide variety of seeds.
Soy, non-GMO	Tofu (all varieties, plain or smoked), tempeh (plain)	While soy products (such as faux meats) are not allowed in phase two, soy proteins, such as tofu and plain tempeh, are recommended. Have a 3- to 4-ounce serving up to three times a day.
Vegetables	Asparagus, broccoli, Brussels sprouts, cabbage, carrots, cauliflower, celery, chard, collard greens, cucumber, eggplant, garlic, ginger, green beans, kale, leeks, lettuce, mushrooms, onions, peppers, radicchio, radishes, sea vegetables, snap peas, snow peas, spinach, summer squash, tomato, zucchini	Fill at least half your plate with one or more of these vegetables. Add sea vegetables to your meals at least three times per week. Sea vegetables provide minerals such as iodine and iron that can be difficult to obtain on a plant-based diet. They also aid digestion and add flavor.

Table 5. Foods to avoid on phase two

Type of Food	Foods to Avoid
Beverages	Anything sweetened, including alcohol, juices, nondairy milk
Fats and Oils	Margarine and any items that contain hydrogenated oil or partially hydrogenated oil, canola oil, corn oil, safflower oil, soybean oil, sunflower oil, vegetable oil
Fruit	All fruits (except avocado, coconut, lemon, lime)
Grains	Short-grain rice, white rice, any processed grains (such as baked goods, flour, or pasta), any refined grains (such as white rice)
Other proteins	Any plant-based meat alternatives, such as veggie burgers, ground round, chick'n, or veggie dogs
Vegetables	High-starch vegetables, such as potato, rutabaga, sweet potato, turnip, winter squash, yam

Table 6. The daily meal plan on phase two

Type of Food	Recommendations
Fats/Oils	One 1-ounce serving of avocado, nuts/seeds, or oil per meal
Grains	1 cup cooked grains, up to twice daily
Protein	3 to 4 ounces tofu or tempeh, or ½ cup cooked legumes per meal
Snacks	Include a balance of fat, protein, and carbohydrates to keep you satisfied
Vegetables	At least half your plate at every meal

Phase Two Breakfast Ideas

Chia Pudding: Soak ¼ cup chia seeds in 1 cup unsweetened nondairy milk in the refrigerator for 8 to 12 hours. Add a sprinkle of pumpkins seeds or hemp seeds and ground cinnamon to taste.

Green Smoothie: Blend ½ avocado, ½ cucumber, 1 tablespoon almond butter, 1 tablespoon hemp seeds, ½ to 1 cup baby spinach, dash ground cinnamon, ½ to 1 cup unsweetened almond milk, and ½ cup ice cubes until smooth. **Variation:** Add ground ginger, ground cloves, and/or ground nutmeg in place of or in addition to the cinnamon, or swap the almond butter for peanut butter or tahini.

Overnight Oats: Soak ½ cup rolled oats in ½ cup unsweetened nondairy milk in the refrigerator for 8 to 12 hours. In the morning, stir in 1 tablespoon sunflower seed butter, sprinkle with ground nutmeg, and top with additional nondairy milk.

Tofu Skillet: 3 ounces tofu, tempeh, or chickpeas cooked in extra-virgin olive oil and served over sautéed kale, with a side of sliced fresh tomato. Add any approved vegetables in table 4 (page 33).

Phase Two Lunch and Dinner Ideas

Burrito Bowl: Crumble 3 ounces tempeh or tofu in a skillet and season with ground coriander, ground cumin, minced garlic, dried oregano, paprika, ground pepper, and salt to taste. Add chopped onion, diced red and green bell peppers, and a few handfuls of chopped leafy greens. Sauté until tender and serve over 1 cup cooked long-grain brown rice or sorghum. Garnish with diced fresh tomato and avocado and a spritz of lime juice.

The Big Salad: Load up a large bowl with dark leafy salad greens, any of the approved vegetables in table 4 (page 33), and a serving of tofu, tempeh, or legumes. Add ½ cup cooked whole grains for a more filling meal. Sprinkle with Crunchy Chickpeas (page 45) for a crouton alternative.

The Warm Salad: If it's too cold to enjoy a crisp, chilled salad, try the same ingredients as in The Big Salad but warm them instead. Sauté the greens in a skillet until they're just wilted, and roast the remaining vegetables on a baking sheet until crisp and golden. Toss the veggies with your favorite olive oil and dark balsamic vinegar or the dressing from Shredded Vegetable Salad (page 44) and serve warm.

Simple Stir-Fry: Sauté any approved vegetables (see table 4, page 33) in a skillet, then splash with one of the flavor combinations below. Serve with 1 cup of approved grains.

- Ground black pepper, minced hot chiles, ground cumin, and lemon or lime juice
- Lemon juice and fresh or dried oregano
- Peanut butter, grated fresh ginger, reduced-sodium tamari, and lime juice
- Reduced-sodium tamari and sesame oil
- Tahini, lemon juice, and minced garlic

Tomato Vegetable Soup: Use the recipe for Classic Tomato Soup (page 43) and add any other approved vegetables, grains, and legumes (see table 4, page 33) to the pot. Make a big batch and store it in single-serving portions in the freezer for a quick lunch or dinner.

Phase Two Snacks

- Any approved vegetables (see table 4, page 33) with ⅓ cup homemade hummus or bean dip
- Any approved vegetables with 2 tablespoons peanut or nut butter, or 1 ounce nuts
- ½ cup Anything Goes Granola (page 42)
- ½ cup Crunchy Chickpeas (page 45)
- ½ sliced avocado and alfalfa sprouts rolled in 2 sheets of nori
- Chia Pudding (page 34)
- Green beans tossed with olive oil and roasted in the oven until tender-crisp

Phase Three

Congratulations on making it this far! Although phase three is a maintenance plan for the rest of your life, there are still a few guidelines and limitations. As you move through the weeks, you'll see what works for you and gauge how much you can consume without slipping back into those peaks of sugar highs and crashes.

During phase three you'll be able to add back a number of foods that were off limits in phase two. Some items are still not advised, while others should be consumed in limited amounts. Table 7 lists what you can enjoy, along with recommendations for serving sizes.

Table 7. Foods to enjoy in phase three

Type of Food	Foods Allowed	Notes
Beverages (no sugar added)	Coffee, sparkling water, low-sodium club soda, unsweetened nondairy beverages, unsweetened tea	Any sweetened or artificially sweetened beverages are off limits during this phase. If you regularly indulge in sodas, juices, and other sugary beverages, take ten days to wean yourself off them before starting on phase two of the detox.
Fruits	All fruits	Fruits are limited because of their high sugar content.
Grains, whole	Amaranth, long-grain brown rice, Kamut, quinoa, sorghum, spelt, steel-cut oats, old-fashioned rolled oats, teff, wild rice All whole grains and processed whole grains (such as bread or baked goods) using 100 percent whole-grain flour	Have up to 1 cup of cooked whole grains twice a day.
Legumes	All legumes (beans, lentils, and peas)	Have up to ½ cup of cooked legumes per meal.
Nuts and Sugar-Free Nut Butters	Almonds, Brazil nuts, cashews, coconut, hazelnuts, peanuts, pecans, pistachios, walnuts	Look for nut butters that only contain nuts and salt. Limit nuts to a 1-ounce serving about three times a day and choose from a wide variety of nuts.

Oils	Avocado oil, coconut oil, extra-virgin olive oil, flaxseed oil, nut oils (almond, macadamia, walnut), pumpkin seed oil, sesame oil	There are no maximums for fats and oils on the detox, but be mindful of how much you are taking in. About one-eighth of your meals and snacks should contain some sort of fat, which includes avocado, coconut, seeds, and nuts.
Seeds and Seed Butters (no sugar added)	Chia, flax, hemp, pumpkin, sesame, sunflower, tahini	Look for seed butters that only include seeds and salt. Limit seeds to a 1-ounce serving about three times a day and choose from a wide variety of seeds.
Soy, non-GMO	Tofu (all varieties, plain or smoked), tempeh (plain)	While soy products (such as faux meats) are not recommended in phase three, soy proteins, such as tofu and plain tempeh are. Have a 3- to 4-ounce serving up to three times a day.
Vegetables	Asparagus, broccoli, Brussels sprouts, cabbage, carrots, cauliflower, celery, chard, collard greens, cucumber, eggplant, garlic, ginger, green beans, kale, leeks, lettuce, mushrooms, onions, parsnips, peppers, potatoes, pumpkin, radicchio, radishes, rutabaga, sea vegetables, snap peas, snow peas, spinach, summer squash, sweet potatoes, tomato, turnips, winter squash, yams, zucchini	Fill at least half your plate with one or more of these vegetables. Add sea vegetables to your meals at least three times per week. Sea vegetables provide minerals such as iodine and iron that can be difficult to obtain on a plant-based diet. They also aid digestion and add flavor.

Additional Phase Three Recommendations
Vegetables
All vegetables listed in phase two should be enjoyed freely in phase three and comprise 50 percent of any meal. The following starchy vegetables have the following recommendations:
- Beet root, parsnip, pumpkin, turnip, sweet potato, winter squash, potato: ¾ cup mashed
- Corn, green peas: ½ cup

As these vegetables are reintroduced, include them in grain-free and legume-free meals that include tofu or tempeh. This will help you to assess the effects of these higher-sugar foods on your symptoms.

Fruit
All fruit can be enjoyed during phase three. However, some fruits should be more limited than others because of their higher sugar content, such as mango, melon, papaya, pineapple, and watermelon. Eat these fruits a maximum of once a week, and limit the portion size to 1 cup of chunks.

Start with adding one serving of fruit and work your way up to a maximum of three servings per day, following these guidelines:
- Whole fruits, such as apples, bananas, nectarines, oranges, and peaches, should be 1 small fruit per serving.
- One serving of berries equals a total of ¾ cup.
- Small fruits, such as apricots, kiwi, plums, and tangerines, should be 2 small fruits.
- Dried fruit should be consumed in very small amounts, about 2 tablespoons of the chopped fruit per serving.

Grains
Grain servings for phase three are the same as in phase two, but processed grains, such as bread, pasta, and flour, are allowed if they contain 100 percent of the whole grain. Use the label-reading techniques on page 8 to find the best products available. Prioritize whole grains and keep processed grains to a maximum of one serving per day.

Everything in Moderation

The foods you'll need to avoid during phase three are minimal. Mostly, just use your common sense while bearing in mind the following guidelines:

- If you don't recognize the ingredient or can't pronounce it, or the product contains preservatives, food coloring, or artificial sweeteners, it should be avoided.
- If the ingredient label contains any of the words for sugar as noted in the list on page 8, and you are still struggling with sugar cravings or health concerns, that product should be avoided. If you are comfortable with your current health situation and don't feel that you still have a reliance on sugar, enjoy that product infrequently.
- Choose whole foods rather than packaged foods as often as possible.
- For an average day, eat up to 3 servings of legumes, 2 servings of whole grains, plenty of nonstarchy vegetables, 1 or 2 servings of starchy vegetables, high-quality fats (including avocado, nuts, oils, and seeds), and as many spices and herbs as you like.
- Keep sugary and processed foods out of the house to avoid temptation, or buy single-serving sizes for when the time is right.
- Eat a wide variety of foods: don't limit yourself to one kind of legume or grain or the same vegetables day after day. Experiment and explore new tastes!

Phase Three Meal Options

Unlike phase two, where your options are a little more limited, phase three has nearly no barriers for experimentation. Sometimes substitutes may be needed if you're following a recipe with ingredients that aren't recommended. Look for recipes with no added sugar in the ingredient list and that don't contain high-sugar processed foods as flavoring agents (such as ketchup). Use the ideas listed in Simple Swaps (page 31) to reconstruct a recipe, or try your hand at creating your own taste combinations in the kitchen. You can't go wrong with fresh herbs, spices, and whole foods as ingredients—if you like what's going in, chances are, you'll love the end result. The recipes on pages 42 through 45 include some staples to help you get started.

Conclusion

Whether you haven't started your detox journey yet, are picking up this guidebook for a second time around, or are simply curious about the process, remember that getting rid of excess sugar in your diet is taking a major step toward improving both your mental and physical health. If you've completed the detox, revisit the questions in the introduction on page 4 and see if your answers have changed. You may be surprised to find that your yeses have turned to nos now that you've established a new, healthy lifestyle and a more positive approach toward eating.

Recipes

Be sure to see the variations that follow each recipe in this section for even more ideas. Additional basic recipes can be found on pages 34 to 36.

Anything Goes Granola

Makes 4 servings

This all-purpose granola is the perfect breakfast or snack. It can also be made into a savory version for a delicious salad topper.

- 2 tablespoons coconut oil, melted
- 2 tablespoons extra-virgin olive oil
- 2 tablespoons unsweetened nondairy milk
- ¼ teaspoon vanilla extract
- 3 cups old-fashioned rolled oats or buckwheat groats
- ½ cup chopped walnuts
- ¼ cup unsweetened large-flaked coconut
- ¼ cup ground flaxseeds
- ¼ cup raw pumpkin seeds
- ½ teaspoon ground cinnamon
- ¼ teaspoon salt

Preheat the oven to 400 degrees F. Line a rimmed baking sheet with parchment paper.

Put the coconut oil, olive oil, milk, and vanilla extract in a saucepan. Heat over medium-low heat until warm. Whisk well to combine.

Put the oats, walnuts, coconut, flaxseeds, pumpkin seeds, cinnamon, and salt in a large bowl. Add the coconut oil mixture and stir until evenly distributed and well combined. Spread the mixture on the lined baking sheet. Bake for 12 minutes. Stir. Bake for 5 to 10 minutes longer, until fragrant and starting to crisp. The granola will get crunchier as it cools. Cool completely before storing.

Variations

- For phase three, add ¼ cup of chopped dried fruit, such as raisins, unsweetened cranberries, or chopped dates, after baking.
- For a savory snack or salad sprinkle, omit the cinnamon and add 1 teaspoon of curry powder.
- Replace the walnuts and pumpkin seeds with equal amounts of any other nuts or seeds.

Classic Tomato Soup

Makes 4 servings

Use this recipe as a starting point for your own signature soup by adding the herbs, spices, whole grains, and legumes of your choice.

2 tablespoons extra-virgin olive oil
1 yellow onion, diced
2 cloves garlic, minced
Salt
Freshly ground black pepper
1 can (28 ounces) whole peeled tomatoes in juice, crushed with a fork, or 3 to 4 cups peeled and chopped fresh tomatoes
1½ cups low-sodium vegetable broth
⅓ cup unsweetened nondairy milk or additional vegetable broth

Heat the oil in a medium soup pot over medium-low heat. Add the onion and cook, stirring occasionally, until soft, about 10 minutes. Add the garlic and cook, stirring almost constantly, until fragrant, about 2 minutes. Add a sprinkle of salt and pepper.

Increase the heat to medium and add the tomatoes and their juice. Cook until the tomatoes are softened and hot, about 10 minutes. Add the broth and simmer for 10 minutes. Process the soup with an immersion blender or in batches in a regular blender until smooth. Stir in the milk and cook, stirring frequently, until the soup is hot. Season with additional salt and pepper to taste.

Variations

- Add ⅓ cup of cooked or canned chickpeas or white beans or cubed soft tofu.
- Add Mexican flair by seasoning with ground cumin and chili powder to taste.
- Add Indian flavor by seasoning with curry powder, garam masala, and ground turmeric to taste.
- Add Italian flavor by seasoning with basil, marjoram, oregano, and rosemary to taste.
- For a Thai twist, use lite coconut milk instead of the nondairy milk and stir in 1 teaspoon of vegan red curry paste.

Shredded Vegetable Salad

Makes 4 servings

Salads don't have to be built on lettuce or be served only in summer. This warm shredded salad will satisfy you even on chilly nights. Try the tahini dressing drizzled over roasted vegetables, stirred into Classic Tomato Soup (page 43) for added richness, or served as a dipping sauce for carrots and celery.

Shredded Salad
- 2 tablespoons extra-virgin olive oil
- 1 large red onion, thinly sliced
- 8 cups coarsely chopped kale, packed
- 2 large carrots, shredded
- 2 large turnips, shredded (for phase three only)

Tahini Dressing
- ½ cup tahini
- 1 large lemon, juiced
- 2 tablespoons capers
- 1 clove garlic, minced
- Warm water, as needed
- Salt
- Freshly ground black pepper

To make the salad, put the oil in a large skillet and heat over medium heat. When hot, add the onion and cook, stirring frequently, until it starts to soften, about 5 minutes. Add the kale, turn off the heat, and cook the kale in the hot skillet, stirring constantly, until it starts to wilt and soften.

Transfer the kale mixture into a large serving bowl. Add the carrots and turnips, if using. Season with salt and pepper to taste.

To make the dressing, put the tahini, lemon juice, capers, and garlic in a measuring cup or small bowl. Whisk until smooth, adding warm water as needed to make a thick dressing. Season with salt and pepper to taste and whisk until well incorporated. Add the dressing to the kale mixture and toss until evenly distributed. Let stand for 30 minutes before serving. Serve at room temperature.

Variations
- Try any other leafy greens that you like, such as Swiss chard, spinach, or even shredded cabbage or Brussels sprouts. Use what you have on hand and what is in season.
- If you're on phase three, add a shredded tart apple to the cooked kale for a bit of tang and natural sweetness.
- If you prefer everything raw, don't cook the kale but make the salad a day in advance so the kale and onions have a chance to soften naturally and mellow.

Crunchy Chickpeas

Makes 4 servings

Try these high-protein beans as a tasty snack or garnish, or as a replacement for croutons on your favorite salads.

> 2 cups cooked or canned chickpeas, rinsed, drained, and patted dry
> 2 tablespoons oil (see variations)
> ½ teaspoon salt
> Spices (see variations)

Preheat the oven to 350 degrees F. Put the chickpeas in a large bowl. Toss with the oil until well coated. Add the salt and spices of your choice and toss until evenly distributed.

Spread the chickpeas in a single layer on a baking sheet. Roast for 50 to 60 minutes, shaking the pan every 20 minutes, until the chickpeas are very firm and dry. They will become crunchier as they cool.

Spice Variations

- Asian: 1 teaspoon ground ginger and ¼ teaspoon garlic powder (use sesame oil)
- Greek: 2 teaspoons dried oregano and ½ teaspoon garlic powder (use olive oil)
- Indian: 1 teaspoon ground coriander, 1 teaspoon curry powder, and 1 teaspoon ground turmeric (use melted coconut oil)
- Italian: 1 tablespoon Italian seasoning (use olive oil)
- Smoky: 2 teaspoons smoked paprika (use olive oil)
- Sweet and Spicy: 1 teaspoon cayenne and 1 teaspoon ground cinnamon (use melted coconut oil)
- Thai: 1 teaspoon vegan red curry paste, whisked with the oil (use melted coconut oil)

Resources

Glycemic Index
World's Healthiest Foods
http://goo.gl/n5pRCo

Glycemic Index Database
glycemicindex.com

References

American Heart Association. 2016. "Added Sugars." February 9. http://goo.gl/Xf4u25.

Bellisle, F. and A. Drewnowski. 2007. "Intense Sweeteners, Energy Intake, and the Control of Body Weight." *European Journal of Clinical Nutrition* 61(6): 691–700. doi:10.1038/sj.ejcn.1602649.

Euromonitor International. 2014. "The Sugar Backlash and Its Effects on Global Consumer Markets." http://goo.gl/I0ZqVp.

Fagherazzi G., et al. 2013. "Consumption of Artificially and Sugar-sweetened Beverages and Incident Type 2 Diabetes in the Etude Epidemiologique aupres des femmes de la Mutuelle Generale de l'Education Nationale: European Prospective Investigation into Cancer and Nutrition Cohort." *American Journal of Clinical Nutrition* 97(3): 517–23. doi:10.3945/ajcn.112.050997.

Ferdman, Roberto A. 2015. "Where People around the World Eat the Most Sugar and Fat," *Washington Post*, February 5. https://goo.gl/fpoBQN.

US Department of Agriculture Office of Communications. 2003. "Profiling Food Consumption in America." Chap. 2 in *Agriculture Fact Book 2001–2002*. 13–21. Washington, DC: US Government Printing Office.

World Health Organization. 2015. "WHO Calls on Countries to Reduce Sugars Intake among Children and Adults." March 4. http://goo.gl/FXL36M.

Yang, Q, et al. 2014. "Added Sugar Intake and Cardiovascular Disease Mortality among US Adults." *JAMA Internal Medicine* 174(4): 516–524. doi:10.1001/jamainternmed.2013.13563.

About the Author

Ann Eugene is a Canadian author who thrives on encouraging others to embrace life fully. Her experience as a fitness instructor and health professional has provided her with the opportunity to help others through exercise and nutrition. She is devoted to creating easily accessible lifestyle changes using a plant-based protocol that eschews deprivation.

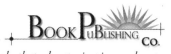

books that educate, inspire, and empower

All titles in the **Live Healthy Now** series are only **$5.95!**

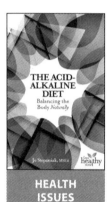
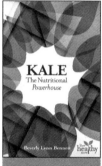
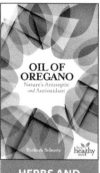
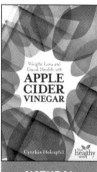

HEALTH ISSUES	HEALTHY FOODS	HERBS AND SUPPLEMENTS	NATURAL SOLUTIONS
GLUTEN-FREE Success Strategies	**KALE** The Nutritional Powerhouse	**OLIVE LEAF EXTRACT** The Mediterranean Healing Herb	Weight Loss and Good Health with **APPLE CIDER VINEGAR**
A Holistic Approach to **ADHD**	Enhance Your Health with **FERMENTED FOODS**	**AROMATHERAPY** Essential Oils for Healing	Healthy and Beautiful with **COCONUT OIL**
Understanding **GOUT**	**GREEN SMOOTHIES:** The Easy Way to Get Your Greens	The Pure Power of **MACA**	The Weekend **DETOX**
WHEAT BELLY– Is Modern Wheat Causing Modern Ills?	**PALEO** Smoothies		Improve Digestion with **FOOD COMBINING**
The **ACID-ALKALINE** Diet	Refreshing Fruit and Vegetable **SMOOTHIES**		The Healing Power of **TURMERIC**

Interested in other health topics or healthy cookbooks? See our complete line of titles at **BookPubCo.com** or order directly from:
Book Publishing Company • PO Box 99 • Summertown, TN 38483 • 1-888-260-8458